USAGE GUIDE ON CLOBETASOL PROPIONATE

Effective Treatment Strategies for Inflammatory and Autoimmune Skin Conditions

Dr. Rembert Vijay

Contents

CHAPTER ONE 3
    Introduction 3
    Mechanism of Action 7
    Administration and Dosage 18
    Comparison to Other Corticosteroids 24
    Adverse Effects and Complications 30
CHAPTER TWO 37
    Special Populations 37
    Clinical Studies and Evidence 41
    Lifestyle and Management Tips 46
    Future Directions and Research 50
    Research and Trials in Progress 53
    Patient Resources and Support 56
THE END 62

CHAPTER ONE

Introduction

What is Clobetasol Propionate?

Clobetasol propionate is a synthetic corticosteroid developed for treating severe inflammatory diseases, primarily of the skin. Being in

Class I corticosteroids, it is at the highest potency class and exerts marked anti-inflammatory and immunosuppressive activity. It comes in different topical preparations like creams, ointments, gels, and sprays.

Historical Background

Designed and cleared in the late 1980s, clobetasol propionate represented an advance in dermatological treatment. Before its introduction, severe skin conditions had been treated with less effective therapy, and clobetasol was a stronger medication for the management of conditions resistant to former therapies.

Purpose of the Book

This book on clobetasol propionate describes the mechanisms of action, clinical uses, administration, and management. Topics include: This is a comprehensive resource for the health professional and the patient who must understand this powerful drug in intimate detail.

Mechanism of Action

Molecular Mechanisms

Clobetasol propionate is similar in action to cortisol, a naturally occurring hormone from the adrenal glands. It binds with corticosteroid receptors that are part of the cytoplasm of a target cell. The receptor steroid complex moves into the cell nucleus and influences the transcription of genes participating in the inflammatory and immune processes.

Corticosteroid Receptors

Type I, or mineralocorticoid receptors, predominantly influence electrolyte and fluid equilibrium, but are also involved in the inflammatory process. Type II, or glucocorticoid receptors, are implicated directly in antiinflammatory and immunosuppressive action. The highly potent clobetasol propionate has a high affinity for type II receptors.

Gene transcription modulation: The receptor

steroid complex binds to glucocorticoid response elements on DNA and thereby promotes or inhibits the transcription of various genes that code for proinflammatory molecules involved in inflammation. Cytokine Production: It reduces the production of proinflammatory cytokines such as TNFalpha, IL1, and IL6. Cell Proliferation: Inhibition of the proliferation of T cells and other immune cells, which are involved in the inflammatory process.

Psoriasis: A chronic skin disorder characterized by scaly, itchy patches. Clobetasol reduces inflammation, scaling, and discomfort. It is usually prescribed for disease that is unresponsive to less potent agents.

Eczema (Atopic Dermatitis): An allergic reaction causing redness and itching of the skin. Clobetasol decreases the redness and itching of the skin, with flare ups in many cases being controlled.

Contact Dermatitis: This results from an active contact allergen or irritant. Clobetasol relieves inflammation and symptoms such as itching and swelling.

Lichen Planus: This is an autoimmune disease characterized by purplish, itchy bumps. Clobetasol decreases inflammation and enhances the appearance of the skin.

Autoimmune Disorders

Systemic Lupus Erythematosus (SLE): Clobetasol formulations are recommended for skin rashes and lesions that occur due to lupus.

Bullous Pemphigoid: A disease that is characterized by large blisters and itching. Clobetasol is useful in diminishing inflammation and promoting the healing process.

Other Clinical Uses

Scalp Disorders: Clobetasol is indicated for inflammatory scalp disorders, including seborrheic dermatitis and psoriasis of the scalp.

Nail Disorders: Useful in inflammatory nail disorders, especially where conventional treatments fail.

Administration and Dosage

Forms and Preparations

Creams: Indicated for nonocclusive use. Suitable for general skin use.

Ointments: Thicker, more occlusive product. Suitable for dry or thickened skin areas.

Gels: Non Greasy formulation, good for hairy areas or when a less oily product is desired.

Sprays: Convenient application on large or difficult to reach areas such as the scalp.

Application Techniques

Cream/Ointment: Apply a thin layer to the affected area once or twice daily. Occlusive dressings should not be used unless specifically instructed by a healthcare provider.

Gel: A thin layer to the affected area once to twice daily; the gel should be thinly spread and rubbed in until it disappears.

Spray: The can should be held 6 inches from the skin. Spray on the affected area evenly, avoiding inhaling the spray or getting it in your eyes.

Dosage Recommendations and Adjustments

Initial Treatment: Generally involves more frequent

applications to rapidly achieve control of the condition.

Maintenance Therapy: Reduce frequency once symptoms are controlled in order to avoid the potential side effects. In general, treatment duration must be limited to 24 continuous weeks.

Adjustment for Special Populations: Adjustments in

dosage and frequency in pediatric patients and patients with sensitive skin.

Comparison to Other Corticosteroids

Potency and Efficacy

Clobetasol vs. Betamethasone: Clobetasol is stronger than betamethasone and, while it may be more effective in severe conditions, it bears the added risk of developing side effects.

Clobetasol vs. Triamcinolone: Triamcinolone is a corticosteroid of medium potency but has a much wider margin of safety, perhaps being much less effective in more serious skin conditions compared to clobetasol.

Comparison of Side Effects

Clobetasol: Increased risk of side effects due to more potent strength as compared to other corticosteroids of lower strengths, such as thinning of the skin and systemic absorption.

Betamethasone and Triamcinolone: Generally

have fewer adverse effects but are less effective during flare ups.

Clinical DecisionMaking

Choice of Therapy: Corticosteroid selection depends upon disease severity, site of application, and patient health conditions. For grave diseases, clobetasol treatment is commonly used despite all the risks associated with it.

Adverse Effects and Complications

Common Adverse Effects

Skin Thinning: Long Term administration may lead to skin atrophy, which injures easily and is bruised.

Striae (Stretch Marks): From changes in skin elasticity.

These occur especially in those areas where the administration of the drug is frequently applied.

Telangiectasia: Small blood vessels appear on the surface of the skin. This usually results from skin thinning.

Serious Adverse Reactions

Systemic Absorption: With extensive use or under occlusion, systemic absorption may occur, which can cause adrenal suppression and other systemic effects.

Hypopigmentation: Skin lightening in areas of application is possible, more apparent in people of color.

Secondary Infections: Bacterial, fungal, or viral infections are also possible due to the immunosuppressive nature of the medication.

LongTerm Risks and Management

Adrenal Suppression: Long Term therapy can cause

suppression, as a result of which the body may not be able to synthesize corticosteroids naturally. It will, therefore, always be necessary to keep patients under regular medical supervision while on long term treatment.

Growth Suppression in Children: Long Term

treatment may lead to growth suppression in children; hence, the length of such treatment must be kept as short as possible.

Contraindications and Drug Interactions

Hypersensitivity: Contraindicated in patients

with a history of hypersensitivity to clobetasol propionate or any of the components of the formulation.

Drug Interactions: No significant systemic interactions noted; caution is advised when used in conjunction with other agents affecting skin integrity or immune function.

CHAPTER TWO

Special Populations

Pediatric Use

Safety and Efficacy: Clobetasol is effective in

pediatric patients; however, close monitoring is required due to the potential for growth suppression and skin sensitivity.

Dosing Adjustments: Doses for pediatrics are typically lower with shorter durations of action.

Pregnancy: Category C; use only if clearly needed and avoid extensive use. Fetal risks should be weighed, and alternatives should be considered.

Lactation: Clobetasol is excreted in breast milk; avoid applications to the breast in a way that would minimize exposure to the infant. Consult healthcare professionals for advice.

Elderly Patients

AgeRelated Considerations
The skin of elderly patients may be very sensitive, and they are at an increased risk for many side effects. The dosage is generally lower and

treatment, including skin thinning and systemic absorption.

Comparative Safety: Compared to weaker corticosteroids, the safety profile for clobetasol is higher and hence requires more scrutiny and management.

Comparative Effectiveness

efficacy in grave conditions but with increased risks.

Safety and Tolerability

LongTerm Studies: Long Term trials, while stating the efficacy, stress that it needs very careful monitoring because of the risks associated with this modality of inflammatory conditions of the skin, symptoms and quality of life have been greatly improved by clobetasol propionate.

Comparative Studies: Comparisons in which clobetasol is pitted against other corticosteroids in a placebo controlled manner have demonstrated greater the duration of treatment shorter.

Clinical Studies and Evidence

Research on Efficacy

Clinical Trials Highly effective treatment in severe

Potency Comparison: Trials that compare clobetasol with other high potency corticosteroids reveal its efficacy in grave conditions but also point out its higher propensity for side effects.

Lifestyle and Management Tips

Minimizing Side Effects

Application Techniques: Apply a thin layer to the affected area. Avoid overapplication. Go easy on it to minimize the chances of side effects.

Avoid occlusive dressings unless instructed by a healthcare professional to avoid excessive absorption.

Monitoring and FollowUp

Long Term followup is crucial in patients receiving clobetasol therapy. Through regular followup, one will be aware of the aftereffects of treatment and its efficacy. Treatment may have to be adjusted depending on clinical response and side effects. Consider conversion to less potent corticosteroid for long term management.

Patient Education and Support

Inform the patients about the correct application mode, potential side effects, and compliance with prescribed dosages.

Refer the patient to available support groups and professional counseling as part of dealing with chronic diseases and treatment frustrations.

Future Directions and Research

Emerging Clinical Uses

New Indications: There are a number of inflammatory and autoimmune conditions that are under study for possible application of clobetasol propionate.

New Formulations: Newer formations with greater efficiencies and lesser adverse effects are being prepared.

Recent Developments in Delivery Systems

New Modes of Delivery: Initiation and research into novel delivery systems like microneedle patches and nanocarriers have been undertaken, with a view to maximize the effect with minimal systemic absorption.

Combination Therapies: Combination studies with other therapeutic approaches are being undertaken to find a better response while minimizing the chances of adverse drug reactions.

Research and Trials in Progress

Current Investigations: Overview of current clinical

trials investigating the efficacy and safety of clobetasol propionate in different therapeutic settings.

Future Studies: Among the probable future studies, one may also include investigations determining the optimal dosage schedules, further indications for its use, and the formulation of safer preparations.

Patient Resources and Support

Educational Materials

Patient Information Leaflets: Everything about clobetasol propionate in a nutshell, including how it should be taken, possible side effects, and general safety precautions.

Online Resources: Websites and digital tools that may offer supportive information, reinforcement, and other resources for patients.

Support Groups and Counseling

Patient Support Groups: Organizations and online communities providing support to patients on clobetasol propionate and dealing with chronic skin conditions.

Counseling Services: Availability of psychological services to the patient in light of chronic conditions and the impact of treatment on quality of life.

THE END

www.ingramcontent.com/pod-product-compliance
Lightning Source LLC
Chambersburg PA
CBHW030050230526
45471CB00003B/1023